JULIA A. HAWTHORNE

Less Toxic

Beginners guide to reducing harmful toxins: recipes, suggestions and tips

Copyright © 2024 by Julia A. Hawthorne

All rights reserved. No part of this publication may be reproduced, stored or transmitted in any form or by any means, electronic, mechanical, photocopying, recording, scanning, or otherwise without written permission from the publisher. It is illegal to copy this book, post it to a website, or distribute it by any other means without permission.

Julia A. Hawthorne asserts the moral right to be identified as the author of this work.

Julia A. Hawthorne has no responsibility for the persistence or accuracy of URLs for external or third-party Internet Websites referred to in this publication and does not guarantee that any content on such Websites is, or will remain, accurate or appropriate.

Designations used by companies to distinguish their products are often claimed as trademarks. All brand names and product names used in this book and on its cover are trade names, service marks, trademarks and registered trademarks of their respective owners. The publishers and the book are not associated with any product or vendor mentioned in this book. None of the companies referenced within the book have endorsed the book.

First edition

This book was professionally typeset on Reedsy.
Find out more at reedsy.com

Contents

1	Introduction	1
2	Goal Setting using S.M.A.R.T.	3
3	Dangerous chemicals and harm	5
4	Non toxic recipes for your home	9
5	Non toxic Personal Care Recipes	12
6	Food, Sweetners & Sausage Recipe	16
7	Better bread and flour options plus Recipes	21
8	Conclusion	25
9	Resources	27

1

Introduction

Welcome to Less Toxic: Beginners guide to reducing harmful toxins. My name is Julia Hawthorne and I am extremely excited that you've decided to embark on this new journey of natural living. I am an advocate for clean living and I believe small inexpensive changes can have a big impact on the overall health of your family. With 5 children of my own, I am constantly concerned about the widespread use of harmful chemicals in our everyday products and the rising cost of these products. I remember when I first started asking questions and being concerned about product safety and feeling overwhelmed with information; and not knowing where to start. Maybe that's you and you care of course, but time always seems to be lacking in order to make real change. We'll with you in mind the busy parents that are juggling family, work and life.

I created this guide to help you simply start your journey to a healthier home. I know this information is short and concise however the impact it can have if implemented can be big! Our health is our most valuable asset but for many they wait until issues arise to act. My philosophy is simple. Don't wait for your garden to turn brown before you start watering it. Meaning take care of things while they are thriving in hopes that they will continue to thrive. Many times we wait to make changes and the damage has already been done. That is what prompted me to produce this guide, so that your family could benefit now from a less toxic environment rather than dealing with serious health issues later. Of course in the world in which we live there is no absolute in anything. However, I believe if we do our part we can benefit from healthier lives by simply removing unnecessary toxins.

With this guide you can expect basic information on harmful chemicals, words of encouragement for your new journey, recipes on how to make safe and budget friendly products, suggestions, tips and how to set S.M.A.R.T. goals to assist you on your new endeavor. While the information I provide will be informational and the recipes proven, this resource is not the end all be all of non toxic information. Rather it is a starting point to give you the momentum to push forward and create a more healthy home environment for your family. Now let's get into it!

2

Goal Setting using S.M.A.R.T.

In chapter one we will be briefly discussing goal setting using the acronym **S.M.A.R.T.** Goal setting is not mandatory but I would encourage you to do it because it helps keep you focused. I have found that more success is obtained when setting clear goals and having a defined action plan to aid you in the process. With any transition, at first it might seem difficult to commit when the other path is easier, however with dedication and patience with yourself you will be able to adopt healthier habits for life, instead of only temporary. The acronym **S.M.A.R.T**. stands for Specific, Measurable, Achievable, Relevant and Time based. The meaning of each letter along with a sample goal is below.

- **Specific**: A specific goal is clear and well-defined. It should state precisely what you are trying to accomplish. Determine the what? and why? (*Sample Goal: To live less toxic buy hand making products or buying healthier options. It is what is best for me and my family over the long run*)
- **Measurable**: A measurable goal allows you to track your progress

and assess how you are doing *(Sample Goal: When I go to the grocery store weekly or bi-weekly, I can read the labels on items before I buy them)*
- **Achievable**: An achievable goal is realistic and attainable. It takes into account your resources, constraints, and abilities. It assures that the goal is within reach but challenging. *(Sample Goal: I can start small buy deciding not to purchase any items containing high fructose corn syrup)*
- **Relevant**: A relevant goal is important and aligns with your values, morals or aspiration to do what you feel is right *(Sample Goal: I have to make better buying options or hand make things because my family is my responsibility)*
- **Time-based**: A time-based goals gives you a specific time frame or deadline. It answers the question of when? It helps prevent procrastination. *(Sample Goal: I will not buy anything containing high fructose corn syrup for at least 30 days)*

Now that we've identified the meaning of **S.M.A.R.T.** and understand how to apply it to our specific goals, we can move onto the harmful chemical portion of this guide.

3

Dangerous chemicals and harm

In this chapter we will be discussing the plethora of dangerous chemicals found in our everyday products. These chemicals such as Ammonia, Bleach, Antifreeze, Chlorine, Phthalates, Triclosan, 2-Butoxyethanol, Parabens, Lead, Phosphates, Formaldehyde to name a few. These chemicals have long lasting effects and should not be used in products we use in or on our bodies. These harmful chemicals release dangerous volatile organic compounds known as VOCs. VOCs are produced from chemicals that vaporize at room temperature. VOCs can affect respiratory systems, irritate eyes, cause headaches, allergic reactions, etc. Some products known to contain VOCs are aerosol spray products, cleaning products, air fresheners, chlorine bleach, detergent and dishwashing liquid, dry cleaning chemicals, rug and upholstery cleaners, furniture and floor polish, oven cleaners and the list goes on. All of those items that are used almost daily in our homes. Air fresheners to cover up a bathroom order, or detergent to wash our clothes. While the list is endless the dangers are very real. Next we will take a look at 3 of the most widely spread and used chemicals in our products today.

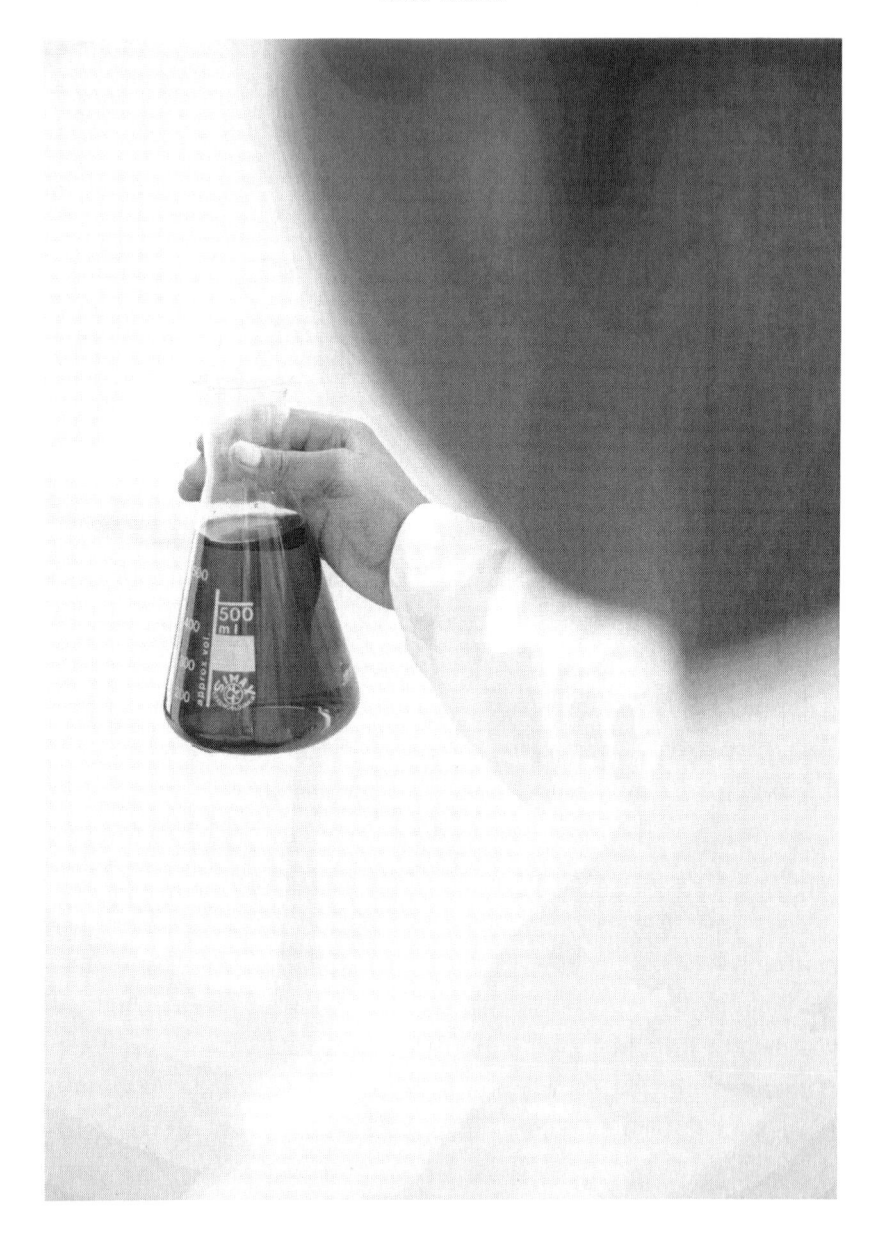

Phthalates can be found in most products that are packaged, produced or delivered using plastic. Which let's be honest! That pretty much covers everything we use religiously daily. Phthalates are endocrine disruptors and are very harmful to humans. Phthalates are chemical compounds that interfere with the normal functioning of the endocrine system and the reproductive and other biological processes regulated by it. Several countries have already adopted regulations or restrictions on the use of phthalates however the U.S. as always is behind the curve! Unfortunately, the U.S. government is controlled and funded by corporations so they don't have the best interest of the people in mind. As long as pockets are getting lined the health and well being of the general public is an afterthought. That's why the system is set up in a way that products can be sold on the market with questionable ingredients and it's up to a consumer to report harm after the harm has already been done! Which is an innocent until proven guilty kind of theory. Which undoubtedly allows multiple harmful chemicals on to the market until there is sufficient evidence that the chemical is indeed harmful. The U.S. has banned less than 20 chemicals in beauty products known to cause harm, while Europe has banned over 1,300. If that information isn't unsettling, then I don't know what is.

Per- and polyfluoroalkyl substances (PFAS) are a group of man-made chemicals that includes PFOA, PFOS, GenX, and many other chemicals. Man-made chemicals are often used as preservatives in foods, beverages, cosmetics and pharmaceuticals. One type of man made chemicals are Parabens. The 4 names used to describe Parabens are methylparaben, propylparaben, butylparaben, and ethylparaben. Parabens are absorbed through the skin or ingested.

While making non toxic items can be budget friendly and quick. Life gets busy and we might lack the time or ingredients to make them. There are several natural companies on the market that produce quality natural products. Just be sure to do your research on the ingredients before purchasing. While the ingredients used may be non toxic each family is different. Some ingredients might not agree with your family, so you might have to try out a few different ones before you can decide on the products that you like. Just as with every new product you introduce into your family, every item does work for everyone so be prepared for some trial and error. Luckily most items have at least a 30 day return window, so if you don't like something. It's your HARD EARNED MONEY, send it back! I am a big believer in customer satisfaction so if you're unhappy the company should make it right! Not little me and you, the consumer.

I have listed a few simple homemade cleaning products using 5 ingredients or less if you are interested in making your own. Or you can scour the internet searching for recipes. I would rather you use the time to make your home less toxic, so I was happy to do the leg work for you!

4

Non toxic recipes for your home

Non toxic laundry detergent using 4 ingredients:

- 1 1/2 cups Sodium Bicarbonate (baking soda)
- 1 1/2 cups Sodium Carbonate (washing soda)
- 1/2 cup Epsom Salt
- 1/4 cup Sea Salt
- 20 drops of Essential Oil (optional)

Place all items in a glass jar and give it a mix. Or you could close the lid and shake it. In order to use, you will need one heaping tablespoon for a regular load and two tablespoons for a larger load. Phthalate, paraben and VOC free.

Non toxic Glass Cleaner using 3 ingredients:

- 2 tablespoons of distilled white vinegar
- 2 Tablespoons of rubbing alcohol
- 2 Cups of water
- 5 drops of essential oil (optional)

Place all ingredients in a spray bottle and give it a little shake to combine. The spray will dissolve grime, grease and dirt leaving a streak free shine. Spray on a microfiber cloth and wipe.

Disinfectant countertop spray:

- ½ cup of vodka (unflavored) or rubbing alcohol
- 1 ½ cups of distilled or previously boiled water
- ½ teaspoon of castile soap
- 7 drops of basil essential oil
- 20 drops of grapefruit essential oil

Combine all ingredients in a 16 oz glass spray bottle and shake. Shake before each use.

Non toxic Fruit and vegetable wash:
(Soaking)

- ¼ cup of white distilled vinegar
- 2 tablespoons salt

In a large mixing bowl or basin pour in vinegar and salt. Swish around with your hand and place fruit and vegetables inside. Let sit and soak for 25-30 minutes. This will draw out bugs, and dirt. It will also remove wax coating. Afterwards, rinse under cold water and pat dry and enjoy or store.

(Quick Cleaning)

- 1 tablespoon fresh lemon juice
- 1 tablespoon baking soda

- 1 cup water

Place ingredients in a glass spray bottle then shake. Spray on produce and let sit 2 to 5 minutes. Then rinse in cold water and pat dry and enjoy or store.

5

Non toxic Personal Care Recipes

Deodorant is an easy way to transition from chemicals. While going natural may take some getting used to, this easy and effective recipe will keep you fresh and dry.

Natural Deodorant:

- ½ cup of baking soda
- ½ cup arrowroot powder or cornstarch (arrowroot powder is best)
- 5 tbsp coconut oil
- 20 drops grapefruit essential oil or another essential oil with antibacterial properties (basil works well also)

Mix baking soda and arrowroot together. Then add the coconut oil and essential oils. Mix well and pour into a clean air-tight container.

Of course home making products are ideal, however there are absolutely instances where you just don't have the time or the energy to make your own. Another option could be researching clean non toxic companies to purchase products from. So, when the time comes and you need products you have already vetted them and trust you are still using a healthier option over traditional. By doing your due diligence beforehand it'll make purchasing products less stressful. While some companies charge a premium for some healthier products, making them yourself is an affordable option. Even switching just a few of the items out for natural ones, could still make a difference. This is not a sprint, but a marathon so no need to get overwhelmed and try to do everything at once. Remember Rome wasn't built in a day, it was built over time and so will healthy habits once you put them into practice. However, you must start somewhere, so small little changes over the next couple weeks or months are okay. Or a drastic change if you're up to it! But please implement some changes, sooner rather than later.

With non toxic toothpaste, there are several great options on the market. Please be sure that it is fluoride free because there is sufficient fluoride found in our tap water. As well as our twice a year fluoride treatment in the dentist office. The everyday use of fluoride in toothpaste could negatively affect your health. Too much fluoride is dangerous and it's best to be cautious. Even though the use of fluoride is still widespread, some dentist offices are committed to being fluoride free. If you are interested in making your own fluoride free toothpaste the process is below. Only 3 ingredients needed for healthy oral hygiene.

All Natural toothpaste:

- ½ cup of room temperature coconut oil
- 4 tablespoons of baking soda
- 15 drops of peppermint essential oil

Mix all ingredients and store in a glass jar. That's it! Homemade non toxic toothpaste that your family will love. I also included a mouthwash recipe for added freshness.

Natural 3 ingredient Mouthwash:

- 2 tablespoons of cloves
- 3 Cinnamon husk sticks
- 8 - 10 oz of boiling water

Take the cloves and cinnamon husks and place in a glass jar. Pour over boiling water and steep overnight. The next day strain and use. Good for up to 2 weeks. This mouthwash will make your breath fresh and has antibacterial properties to prevent the overgrowth of harmful bacteria.

We all need a little moisturizing without the harmful chemicals. Next we have a rich and creamy body butter that your family will love. You can even place it in a cute little container and wrap it with ribbon for a beautiful thoughtful homemade gift.

Homemade body butter/body lotion:

- ¼ cup of Shea Butter
- ¼ cup of Cocoa Butter
- ¼ cup of Coconut Oil
- ¼ cup of Sweet Almond Oil
- 1 tablespoon of arrowroot powder
- 30 drops of Essential Oils (no citrus oils)

Melt the shea butter, cocoa butter, coconut oil and sweet almond oil in a saucepan or double boiler over medium heat. Remove from heat and add essential oils and mix well. Transfer to a mixing bowl and place in fridge to let cool. Allow mixture to cool completely until the oils solidify (overnight is best). *Note: You can place it in the freezer to cool quicker, but be sure to set a timer so you don't forget about it and let it freeze!* Once the mixture is completely cooled, use a hand beater or stand mixer to whip the mixture. Spoon into a clean Mason jar and seal with a lid and voila it's ready to use!

6

Food, Sweetners & Sausage Recipe

Next, we're to my favorite area of expertise by far. Yes, we've covered cleaning, personal care and now let's get into food! Or more specifically sugar and flour substitutes. I will not go so far as to say cane sugar and all purpose white flour are toxic, however I do believe that there are healthier options out there. So, less toxins in our products and our diet are necessary. We will not go into significant detail but we will provide some information that might cause you to pause the next time you're at the grocery store and see cookies, or cereal and even croissants for that matter. Which I cringe to say, because who doesn't love a buttery flaky croissant. OMG!!! My mouth is watering just thinking about it.

If you know me, then you know that baking is near and dear to my heart. I absolutely love making dessert treats, most of which contain bread. I'm talking pies, cakes, cookies, breads, you name it. Especially, if it has fruit and bread together, yum. Over the last couple years I've been alarmed about the amount of sugar in almost everything we eat. While our bodies are now addicted to this sweet flavorful substance the impact of too much of it on our health is clear. Our society as a whole is more unhealthy today than it was 20 years ago and we have 10x the amount of so called healthy options on our grocery shelves. Have you ever asked why that is? Its because most of the population has insulin resistance and one culprit is because of the over consumption of sugar. It's literally in everything! Our drinks, breads, processed foods and even our sauces and condiments contain large amounts of sugar. Also, sugar is used as a preservative in foods and beverages because it prevents microbial growth. So based on that information I can understand why the use of cane sugar is widespread throughout the food industry. While the distinct taste of cane sugar does different from alternatives the switch is still sweet and enjoyable so the adjustment is pretty swift. Like with anything new, it will take some trial and error to find that perfectly sweet balance you crave. But once you find it, you're well on your way! Because it is exciting to experiment with different sweeteners in your desserts. At least that was my experience.

Even though starting a homestead and making everything you consume from scratch would be ideal, is that realistic for most of us? I'm going to say NO! So with that in mind I don't forgo all processed items that I enjoy, but I rather try and limit them so we can be healthier versions of ourselves. Instead of baking an apple tart or pie with cane sugar, I generally opt for coconut sugar, agave or honey. All three are healthier options over white cane sugar that is found in most of our processed, pre packaged grocery items. While on the subject of unhealthy sweeteners lets touch on by far the most widely used and inexpensive form of sweetener which is high fructose corn syrup.

According to Dr. Hyman of the Cleveland Clinic it is cheaper and sweeter than cane sugar and contributes to diabetes, inflammation, high triglycerides and something we call non-alcoholic fatty liver disease. Some other harm that excessive amounts of high fructose corn syrup can cause is increased appetite which promotes obesity, can punch small holes in your intestinal wall causing leaky gut, liver failure and even type 2 diabetes. A great deal of the products marketed to us for our kids as snacks contain high fructose corn syrup. Including fruit snacks, snack cakes, cookies even graham crackers which feels like they should be somewhat wholesome. Our kids will see their friends with these snacks and try to pressure us with their cuteness to buy them, but we have to stand our ground because we know what's best! We don't allow them to make any other important decisions which could cause them harm, so why would we allow them to decide what to put in their bodies when we know certain ingredients cause harm! The data speaks for itself.

So, why with so much information and studies would corporations knowingly put harmful ingredients in their products. The hard reality is because they can! Simply put, If they aren't being regulated to do the right thing, they will always put profits over consumer health which is sad but true. Most of the owners of the corporations don't feed their children with the crap they pedal to our children, so we have to make conscious and informed decisions. Sugar or high fructose corn syrup is included in well over 85% of the food items on the market and has more than 200 different names. It's even in our processed meats. Maple sausages, chicken nuggets and even some hot dogs contain added sweetener. Which is confusing since one would think only maple syrup would be needed to produce a maple flavored sausage. If not, home made items then buy better wholesome items. Simple rule of thumb, when at the grocery store and you read a food label, if you can't pronounce it then you shouldn't buy it! Or if you would question the purpose of putting the ingredient in it, if you were to make it at home. However, making your own sausage is pretty simple and not as scary as you might think. I added a recipe for your convenience that contains no mystery ingredients.

Maple sausage:

- 2 pounds ground turkey
- 1 tablespoon maple sausage
- 2 teaspoons salt
- 1 ½ teaspoons ground black pepper
- 1 ½ teaspoons ground sage
- 1 ½ teaspoons ground thyme
- ½ teaspoon dried fennel
- ½ teaspoon red pepper flakes

Mix together turkey, maple syrup, salt, black pepper, sage, thyme, fennel, and red pepper flakes in a bowl until well combined and refrigerate covered for at least 1 hour to give ingredients time to combine. Shape turkey mixture into patties and you're ready to cook. You can also freeze patties on parchment paper then store in a freezer bag and freeze for quick sausage patties. You could even roll into a log and freeze for later use. Be sure to fully cook until the internal temperature is at least 165 degrees.

While I love to use coconut sugar, agave and honey the healthiest option by far is to sweeten your treats with dates. Which are nature's natural sweetener. Dates are also a good source of antioxidants, mainly carotenoids and phenolics. Dates contain Carbs, Fiber, Protein, Potassium, Magnesium, Copper, Manganese, Iron and Vitamin B6 which prove why it's considered a super food. I love using dates in my peach cobbler especially. I allow them to simmer and release all the sweetness into the peaches while creating a sweet dark syrup. I usually add a little cornstarch (non gmo) or flour to a slurry of the juice to slightly thicken. You will need to remove the pit/seed or buy them already removed. After the peaches are golden and simmered I patiently pick out the dates and use the simmered dates in a smoothie. It adds a wonderful peach flavor. No waste over here!

7

Better bread and flour options plus Recipes

Bread is this girl's best friend! I love a simple piece of sourdough toast with butter. The rich slight tang of the sourdough with the slight salty creaminess of the butter makes a wonderful snack. Speaking of sourdough…………unfortunately there are fake sourdough breads on the market. An authentic sourdough does not contain yeast! I know that sounds strange but it's true. In order for it to be authentic sourdough it uses a 'starter' – a fermented flour and water mixture that contains wild yeast and good bacteria – to rise. Not commercial yeast. Commercial yeast is used to speed up the fermenting process. Authentic sourdough includes good bacteria which is gut healthy. So remember to read the back of the bread package and if you see yeast, it's not real sourdough bread and the extra few bucks is not worth it. Sourdough is a great healthier alternative to traditional breads. If sourdough isn't your thing, you might consider an ancient grain bread. Since breads made with ancient grains are really hard to find, you might make your own with spelt, kamut or millet; of course there are others. While some of these flours might sound strange you could absolutely continue to use regular all purpose flour but please opt for the unbleached option. I have two bread recipes below to try out if you would like to. These recipes are created using spelt flour which is my ancient grain flour of choice. However, you could absolutely substitute another ancient grain flour or all purpose flour of your choice. Just be sure that the ancient grain flour that you choose can be substituted as a 1:1 ration for all purpose flour because all flours are not created equal. As a side bar, I have actually used unbleached all purpose flour for both bread recipes and you absolutely can not tell the difference. So, either choice is fine. Your bread should still come out moist and your crust perfectly flaky provided you follow the directions.

Banana bread

- 2 overly ripe smashed bananas (brown)
- 2 tablespoons of apple sauce or grated apple
- ¼ cup of neutral oil
- ½ cup of milk (plant or regular)
- 2 eggs
- ¼ cup coconut sugar
- ½ cup of honey or agave
- ½ cup of spelt flour (or unbleached all purpose)
- 1 teaspoon of vanilla
- 2 teaspoons baking powder
- ½ teaspoon of salt

Preheat the oven to 325 degrees. Mix wet ingredients: banana, oil, milk eggs, vanilla, honey and set aside. In a separate bowl mix dry ingredients coconut sugar, flour, baking powder and salt. Then combine dry into wet ingredients and mix until incorporated, but do not over mix. Pour into a greased or sprayed bread pan and bake for 50 - 1 hour or until a toothpick comes out clean from the center.

Easy pie crust

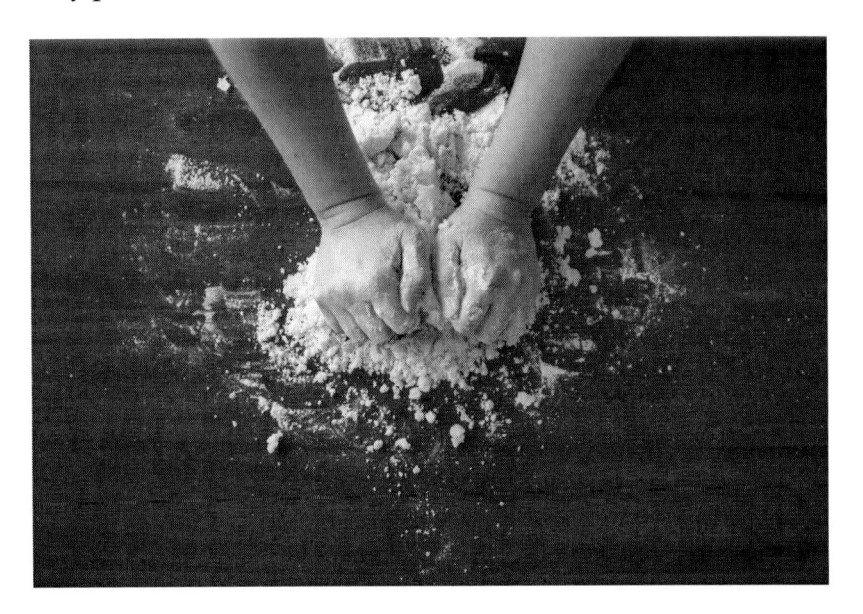

- 1 ½ cups of spelt flour (or unbleached all purpose)
- 2 Tablespoons of coconut sugar
- ½ teaspoon of salt
- One stick of cold butter diced down the middle and then into cubes
- ½ cup of ice cold water

First put flour, coconut sugar and salt into a food processor and pulse a couple times to combine. Then put in the cold butter then pulse to combine. It should be slightly crumbly. Then drizzle in 4 tablespoons of water at a time. Then pulse again until the dough looks slightly crumbly and moist but not wet. You can take a little out to press it into your hands until it slightly sticks together. Pour it on parchment paper and form it into a disk. Use the paper to bring the dough together. Your hands are warm and you don't want to melt the butter. Then place in the fridge for 30 minutes or so to firm up and so the butter can cool again. After 30 minutes or more, roll out and fill with your filling of choice, bake in a 350 degree oven for 20 - 25 minutes and enjoy! I use this recipe as well to make homemade pop tarts. I usually make the filling from scratch using apple and pear, or blueberries, or strawberries but a good quality preserve or store bought pie filling would work just as well. Just be aware of the added sugar content.

8

Conclusion

We've discussed setting **S.M.A.R.T.** goals, harmful chemicals in our cleaning products, personal care products and tips on eating a little healthier. Unfortunately, toxins are all around us and even though there is no 100% way of filtering them all out, we can make better choices that will allow us to have less toxins in our homes and bodies. While pollutants are everywhere we can attempt to mitigate a few by implementing small little changes. I know change is difficulty and the uncertainty of the world is sometimes an overwhelming thought! However, we must stay grounded and remember that we can only do, what we can do. We can't change the world, per say…..but we can change what we spend our money on.

It is sometimes very hard to break from social norms of doing what is convenient especially if everyone is doing it. However, deciding to make healthier changes for your family has to be a personal choice, **not a societal choice**! If we continue down this path of accepting what is normal as right, then we will never break free from the chemical laden products the media, and society pushes on us. If you notice, most marketing is for products that contain harmful chemicals rather than natural holistic ones. The media, and marketing will always follow the trends. Regardless of the undeniable information on the market showing things to be unsafe. With that in mind it is up to us, to break free and stay free as best we can. Of course, we all aren't about to move to the countryside and start a homestead and neither is that a desire of all of us. However, what each and every person can do is make better, more informed choices about the things we allow into our homes and bodies.

Even though there is far more information out there than I could have ever included in this short guide, I sincerely hope you were able to gain some knowledge that will ultimately lead you to think before you buy any products, deemed safe by simply being on grocery shelves. If you decide making homemade products are not for you, hopefully you will at least purchase products that do not contain harmful chemicals to be used by your family. Once again our goal isn't to change the world, but simply to be a little less toxic.

Thank you for purchasing and reading this guide. If you found this guide at all helpful, I would really appreciate it if you left a review on Amazon.

9

Resources

American Lung Association. (n.d.). *Cleaning supplies and household chemicals.* https://www.lung.org/clean-air/indoor-air/indoor-air-pollutants/cleaning-supplies-household-chem

College of Environment, Zhejiang University of Technology, Hangzhou 310032, China & School of Public Health and Preventive Medicine, Monash University, Melbourne 3000, Australia. (2021, May 18). *Phthalates and Their Impacts on Human Health.* https://www.ncbi.nlm.nih.gov. Retrieved January 11, 2023, from https://www.ncbi.nlm.nih.gov/pmc/articles/PMC8157593/

CDC. (2023, December 1). *Parabens Factsheet.* Center for Disease Control and Prevention. Retrieved January 11, 2024, from https://www.cdc.gov/biomonitoring/Parabens_FactSheet.html

Beth, M. (2023, February 25). *DIY Natural Laundry Detergent (without bar soap!).* Boots & Hooves Homestead. https://bootsandhooveshomestead.com/diy-natural-laundry-detergent/

Kielman, J. (2023, October 18). *3 ingredient Homemade natural toothpaste.* Mom 4 Real. https://www.mom4real.com/3-ingredient-homemade-natural-toothpaste/

Wells, K. (2020, May 21). *Easy DIY granite cleaner for naturally clean countertops.* Wellness Mama®. https://wellnessmama.com/natural-home/natural-granite-cleaner/

Homemade vegetable Wash/Preserver that works! (Spray or soak) recipe - Food.com. (2008, April 24). https://www.food.com/recipe/homemade-vegetable-wash-preserver-that-works-spray-or-soak-300387

Sakawsky, A., & Sakawsky, A. (2023, September 12). Homemade whipped body butter recipe - The House & Homestead. *The House & Homestead - Helping you create, grow and live a good life. . . From scratch!* https://thehouseandhomestead.com/homemade-body-butter/

Hansard, J. (2023, January 20). *Homemade deodorant that works.* Simple Green Smoothies. https://simplegreensmoothies.com/homemade-deodorant#wprm-recipe-container-28998

Wambolt, C. (2023, July 31). *Exposure to toxic chemicals in consumer products in the US - Ballard Brief.* Ballard Brief. https://ballardbrief.byu.edu/issue-briefs/exposure-to-toxic-chemicals-in-consumer-products-in-the-united-states

Clinic, C. (2023, November 27). *Avoid the hidden dangers of high fructose corn syrup.* Cleveland Clinic. https://health.clevelandclinic.org/avoid-the-hidden-dangers-of-high-fructose-corn-syrup-video#:~:text=Incr eases%20appetite%2C%20promotes%20obesity&text=%E2%80%9CH igh%20fructose%20corn%20syrup%20also,affects%20over%2090%20

RESOURCES

million%20Americans

Indeed. (n.d.). *SMART Goals: an Acronym for Success.* Indeed.com. https://www.indeed.com/hire/c/info/smart-goals?gclid=Cj0KCQiA wP6sBhDAARIsAPfK_wYm1Ri9xQfPom3Wblvr7ayGyOxgSjh4COo mI1saIc01IjcEdiYYa3IaAqpoEALw_wcB&aceid=&gclsrc=aw.ds

Made in United States
North Haven, CT
10 February 2025